This Medical Journal Belongs to:

_____

If Found, please contact:

Phone Number: _____

E-mail: _____

Medical Diagnosis:

Condition:	Diagnosis Date:

Allergies and Reactions:

Trigger:	Type of Reaction:

Medical Event History

Event:	Date Occurred:

Medication Log:

Medication:	Prescribed By:	Date Started:	Date Ended:

Medication Log:

Medication:	Prescribed By:	Date Started:	Date Ended:

Month:

Appointment Month At a Glance

Month: _____

1	
2	
3	
4	
5	
6	
7	
8	
9	
10	
11	
12	
13	
14	
15	
16	

Appointment Month At a Glance

Month: _____

17	
18	
19	
20	
21	
22	
23	
24	
25	
26	
27	
28	
29	
30	
31	

Pain Tracker

Pain is rated on a 1-5 chart with 1 being the mildest and 5 being the worst. Note any specific pain on the appropriate date.

1	2	3	4	5	6	7
8	9	10	11	12	13	14
15	16	17	18	19	20	21
22	23	24	25	26	27	28
29	30	31				

Fatigue Tracker

Fatigue is rated on a 1-5 chart with 1 being the mildest and 5 being the worst. Note any specific insomnia or difficulty functioning.

1	2	3	4	5	6	7
8	9	10	11	12	13	14
15	16	17	18	19	20	21
22	23	24	25	26	27	28
29	30	31				

Mood Tracker

Mood Key:

1._____   2. _____   3. _____   4._____

5._____

1	2	3	4	5	6	7
8	9	10	11	12	13	14
15	16	17	18	19	20	21
22	23	24	25	26	27	28
29	30	31				

Doctor's Appointment Notes:

Date:

Doctor's Name:

Symptoms to Discuss:

Questions for the Doctor:

Notes from the Appointment:

Doctor's Appointment Notes:

Date:

Doctor's Name:

Symptoms to Discuss:

Questions for the Doctor:

Notes from the Appointment:

Doctor's Appointment Notes:

Date:

Doctor's Name:

Symptoms to Discuss:

Questions for the Doctor:

Notes from the Appointment:

Doctor's Appointment Notes:

Date:

Doctor's Name:

Symptoms to Discuss:

Questions for the Doctor:

Notes from the Appointment:

Doctor's Appointment Notes:

Date:

Doctor's Name:

Symptoms to Discuss:

Questions for the Doctor:

Notes from the Appointment:

Doctor's Appointment Notes:

Date:

Doctor's Name:

Symptoms to Discuss:

Questions for the Doctor:

Notes from the Appointment:

Doctor's Appointment Notes:

Date:

Doctor's Name:

Symptoms to Discuss:

Questions for the Doctor:

Notes from the Appointment:

Month:

Appointment Month At a Glance

Month: _____

1	
2	
3	
4	
5	
6	
7	
8	
9	
10	
11	
12	
13	
14	
15	
16	

Appointment Month At a Glance

Month: _____

17	
18	
19	
20	
21	
22	
23	
24	
25	
26	
27	
28	
29	
30	
31	

Pain Tracker

Pain is rated on a 1-5 chart with 1 being the mildest and 5 being the worst.
Note any specific pain on the appropriate date.

1	2	3	4	5	6	7
8	9	10	11	12	13	14
15	16	17	18	19	20	21
22	23	24	25	26	27	28
29	30	31				

Fatigue Tracker

Fatigue is rated on a 1-5 chart with 1 being the mildest and 5 being the worst. Note any specific insomnia or difficulty functioning.

1	2	3	4	5	6	7
8	9	10	11	12	13	14
15	16	17	18	19	20	21
22	23	24	25	26	27	28
29	30	31				

Mood Tracker

Mood Key:
1._____   2._____   3._____   4._____
5._____

1	2	3	4	5	6	7
8	9	10	11	12	13	14
15	16	17	18	19	20	21
22	23	24	25	26	27	28
29	30	31				

Doctor's Appointment Notes:

Date:

Doctor's Name:

Symptoms to Discuss:	Questions for the Doctor:

Notes from the Appointment:

Doctor's Appointment Notes:

Date:

Doctor's Name:

Symptoms to Discuss:

Questions for the Doctor:

Notes from the Appointment:

Doctor's Appointment Notes:

Date:

Doctor's Name:

Symptoms to Discuss:	Questions for the Doctor:

Notes from the Appointment:

Doctor's Appointment Notes:

Date:

Doctor's Name:

Symptoms to Discuss:	Questions for the Doctor:

Notes from the Appointment:

Doctor's Appointment Notes:

Date:

Doctor's Name:

Symptoms to Discuss:

Questions for the Doctor:

Notes from the Appointment:

Doctor's Appointment Notes:

Date:

Doctor's Name:

Symptoms to Discuss:

Questions for the Doctor:

Notes from the Appointment:

Doctor's Appointment Notes:

Date:

Doctor's Name:

Symptoms to Discuss:

Questions for the Doctor:

Notes from the Appointment:

Month:

Appointment Month At a Glance

Month: _____

1	
2	
3	
4	
5	
6	
7	
8	
9	
10	
11	
12	
13	
14	
15	
16	

Appointment Month At a Glance

Month: _____

17	
18	
19	
20	
21	
22	
23	
24	
25	
26	
27	
28	
29	
30	
31	

Pain Tracker

Pain is rated on a 1-5 chart with 1 being the mildest and 5 being the worst. Note any specific pain on the appropriate date.

1	2	3	4	5	6	7
8	9	10	11	12	13	14
15	16	17	18	19	20	21
22	23	24	25	26	27	28
29	30	31				

Fatigue Tracker

Fatigue is rated on a 1-5 chart with 1 being the mildest and 5 being the worst. Note any specific insomnia or difficulty functioning.

1	2	3	4	5	6	7
8	9	10	11	12	13	14
15	16	17	18	19	20	21
22	23	24	25	26	27	28
29	30	31				

Mood Tracker

Mood Key:

1._____ 2. _____ 3. _____ 4._____

5._____

1	2	3	4	5	6	7
8	9	10	11	12	13	14
15	16	17	18	19	20	21
22	23	24	25	26	27	28
29	30	31				

Doctor's Appointment Notes:

Date:

Doctor's Name:

Symptoms to Discuss:

Questions for the Doctor:

Notes from the Appointment:

Doctor's Appointment Notes:

Date:

Doctor's Name:

Symptoms to Discuss:

Questions for the Doctor:

Notes from the Appointment:

Doctor's Appointment Notes:

Date:

Doctor's Name:

Symptoms to Discuss:

Questions for the Doctor:

Notes from the Appointment:

Doctor's Appointment Notes:

Date:

Doctor's Name:

Symptoms to Discuss:

Questions for the Doctor:

Notes from the Appointment:

Doctor's Appointment Notes:

Date:

Doctor's Name:

Symptoms to Discuss:

Questions for the Doctor:

Notes from the Appointment:

Doctor's Appointment Notes:

Date:

Doctor's Name:

Symptoms to Discuss:

Questions for the Doctor:

Notes from the Appointment:

Doctor's Appointment Notes:

Date:

Doctor's Name:

Symptoms to Discuss:

Questions for the Doctor:

Notes from the Appointment:

Month:

Appointment Month At a Glance

Month: _____

1	
2	
3	
4	
5	
6	
7	
8	
9	
10	
11	
12	
13	
14	
15	
16	

Appointment Month At a Glance

Month: _____

17	
18	
19	
20	
21	
22	
23	
24	
25	
26	
27	
28	
29	
30	
31	

Pain Tracker

Pain is rated on a 1-5 chart with 1 being the mildest and 5 being the worst. Note any specific pain on the appropriate date.

1	2	3	4	5	6	7
8	9	10	11	12	13	14
15	16	17	18	19	20	21
22	23	24	25	26	27	28
29	30	31				

Fatigue Tracker

Fatigue is rated on a 1-5 chart with 1 being the mildest and 5 being the worst. Note any specific insomnia or difficulty functioning.

1	2	3	4	5	6	7
8	9	10	11	12	13	14
15	16	17	18	19	20	21
22	23	24	25	26	27	28
29	30	31				

Mood Tracker

Mood Key:
1._____   2. _____   3. _____   4._____
5._____

1	2	3	4	5	6	7
8	9	10	11	12	13	14
15	16	17	18	19	20	21
22	23	24	25	26	27	28
29	30	31				

Doctor's Appointment Notes:

Date:

Doctor's Name:

Symptoms to Discuss:

Questions for the Doctor:

Notes from the Appointment:

Doctor's Appointment Notes:

Date:

Doctor's Name:

Symptoms to Discuss:

Questions for the Doctor:

Notes from the Appointment:

Doctor's Appointment Notes:

Date:

Doctor's Name:

Symptoms to Discuss:

Questions for the Doctor:

Notes from the Appointment:

Doctor's Appointment Notes:

Date:

Doctor's Name:

Symptoms to Discuss:

Questions for the Doctor:

Notes from the Appointment:

Doctor's Appointment Notes:

Date:

Doctor's Name:

Symptoms to Discuss:

Questions for the Doctor:

Notes from the Appointment:

Doctor's Appointment Notes:

Date:

Doctor's Name:

Symptoms to Discuss:

Questions for the Doctor:

Notes from the Appointment:

Doctor's Appointment Notes:

Date:

Doctor's Name:

Symptoms to Discuss:

Questions for the Doctor:

Notes from the Appointment:

Month:

Appointment Month At a Glance

Month: _____

1	
2	
3	
4	
5	
6	
7	
8	
9	
10	
11	
12	
13	
14	
15	
16	

Appointment Month At a Glance

Month: _____

17	
18	
19	
20	
21	
22	
23	
24	
25	
26	
27	
28	
29	
30	
31	

Pain Tracker

Pain is rated on a 1-5 chart with 1 being the mildest and 5 being the worst. Note any specific pain on the appropriate date.

1	2	3	4	5	6	7
8	9	10	11	12	13	14
15	16	17	18	19	20	21
22	23	24	25	26	27	28
29	30	31				

Fatigue Tracker

Fatigue is rated on a 1-5 chart with 1 being the mildest and 5 being the worst. Note any specific insomnia or difficulty functioning.

1	2	3	4	5	6	7
8	9	10	11	12	13	14
15	16	17	18	19	20	21
22	23	24	25	26	27	28
29	30	31				

Mood Tracker

Mood Key:

1._____ 2._____ 3._____ 4._____

5._____

1	2	3	4	5	6	7
8	9	10	11	12	13	14
15	16	17	18	19	20	21
22	23	24	25	26	27	28
29	30	31				

Doctor's Appointment Notes:

Date:

Doctor's Name:

Symptoms to Discuss:	Questions for the Doctor:

Notes from the Appointment:

Doctor's Appointment Notes:

Date:

Doctor's Name:

Symptoms to Discuss:

Questions for the Doctor:

Notes from the Appointment:

Doctor's Appointment Notes:

Date:

Doctor's Name:

Symptoms to Discuss:

Questions for the Doctor:

Notes from the Appointment:

Doctor's Appointment Notes:

Date:

Doctor's Name:

Symptoms to Discuss:

Questions for the Doctor:

Notes from the Appointment:

Doctor's Appointment Notes:

Date:

Doctor's Name:

Symptoms to Discuss:	Questions for the Doctor:

Notes from the Appointment:

Doctor's Appointment Notes:

Date:

Doctor's Name:

Symptoms to Discuss:

Questions for the Doctor:

Notes from the Appointment:

Doctor's Appointment Notes:

Date:

Doctor's Name:

Symptoms to Discuss:

Questions for the Doctor:

Notes from the Appointment:

Month:

Appointment Month At a Glance

Month: _____

1	
2	
3	
4	
5	
6	
7	
8	
9	
10	
11	
12	
13	
14	
15	
16	

Appointment Month At a Glance

Month: _____

17	
18	
19	
20	
21	
22	
23	
24	
25	
26	
27	
28	
29	
30	
31	

Pain Tracker

Pain is rated on a 1-5 chart with 1 being the mildest and 5 being the worst. Note any specific pain on the appropriate date.

1	2	3	4	5	6	7
8	9	10	11	12	13	14
15	16	17	18	19	20	21
22	23	24	25	26	27	28
29	30	31				

Fatigue Tracker

Fatigue is rated on a 1-5 chart with 1 being the mildest and 5 being the worst. Note any specific insomnia or difficulty functioning.

1	2	3	4	5	6	7
8	9	10	11	12	13	14
15	16	17	18	19	20	21
22	23	24	25	26	27	28
29	30	31				

Mood Tracker

Mood Key:
1._____   2._____   3._____   4._____
5._____

1	2	3	4	5	6	7
8	9	10	11	12	13	14
15	16	17	18	19	20	21
22	23	24	25	26	27	28
29	30	31				

Doctor's Appointment Notes:

Date:

Doctor's Name:

Symptoms to Discuss:	Questions for the Doctor:

Notes from the Appointment:

Doctor's Appointment Notes:

Date:

Doctor's Name:

Symptoms to Discuss:

Questions for the Doctor:

Notes from the Appointment:

Doctor's Appointment Notes:

Date:

Doctor's Name:

Symptoms to Discuss:	Questions for the Doctor:

Notes from the Appointment:

Doctor's Appointment Notes:

Date:

Doctor's Name:

Symptoms to Discuss:	Questions for the Doctor:

Notes from the Appointment:

Doctor's Appointment Notes:

Date:

Doctor's Name:

Symptoms to Discuss:

Questions for the Doctor:

Notes from the Appointment:

Doctor's Appointment Notes:

Date:

Doctor's Name:

Symptoms to Discuss:

Questions for the Doctor:

Notes from the Appointment:

Doctor's Appointment Notes:

Date:

Doctor's Name:

Symptoms to Discuss:

Questions for the Doctor:

Notes from the Appointment:

Month:

Appointment Month At a Glance

Month: _____

1	
2	
3	
4	
5	
6	
7	
8	
9	
10	
11	
12	
13	
14	
15	
16	

Appointment Month At a Glance

Month: _____

17	
18	
19	
20	
21	
22	
23	
24	
25	
26	
27	
28	
29	
30	
31	

Pain Tracker

Pain is rated on a 1-5 chart with 1 being the mildest and 5 being the worst. Note any specific pain on the appropriate date.

1	2	3	4	5	6	7
8	9	10	11	12	13	14
15	16	17	18	19	20	21
22	23	24	25	26	27	28
29	30	31				

Fatigue Tracker

Fatigue is rated on a 1-5 chart with 1 being the mildest and 5 being the worst. Note any specific insomnia or difficulty functioning.

1	2	3	4	5	6	7
8	9	10	11	12	13	14
15	16	17	18	19	20	21
22	23	24	25	26	27	28
29	30	31				

Mood Tracker

Mood Key:
1._____ 2. _____ 3. _____ 4._____
5._____

1	2	3	4	5	6	7
8	9	10	11	12	13	14
15	16	17	18	19	20	21
22	23	24	25	26	27	28
29	30	31				

Doctor's Appointment Notes:

Date:

Doctor's Name:

Symptoms to Discuss:

Questions for the Doctor:

Notes from the Appointment:

Doctor's Appointment Notes:

Date:

Doctor's Name:

Symptoms to Discuss:	Questions for the Doctor:

Notes from the Appointment:

Doctor's Appointment Notes:

Date:

Doctor's Name:

Symptoms to Discuss:

Questions for the Doctor:

Notes from the Appointment:

Doctor's Appointment Notes:

Date:

Doctor's Name:

Symptoms to Discuss:

Questions for the Doctor:

Notes from the Appointment:

Doctor's Appointment Notes:

Date:

Doctor's Name:

Symptoms to Discuss:

Questions for the Doctor:

Notes from the Appointment:

Doctor's Appointment Notes:

Date:

Doctor's Name:

Symptoms to Discuss:

Questions for the Doctor:

Notes from the Appointment:

Doctor's Appointment Notes:

Date:

Doctor's Name:

Symptoms to Discuss:

Questions for the Doctor:

Notes from the Appointment:

Month:

Appointment Month At a Glance

Month: _____

1	
2	
3	
4	
5	
6	
7	
8	
9	
10	
11	
12	
13	
14	
15	
16	

Appointment Month At a Glance

Month: _____

17	
18	
19	
20	
21	
22	
23	
24	
25	
26	
27	
28	
29	
30	
31	

Pain Tracker

Pain is rated on a 1-5 chart with 1 being the mildest and 5 being the worst. Note any specific pain on the appropriate date.

1	2	3	4	5	6	7
8	9	10	11	12	13	14
15	16	17	18	19	20	21
22	23	24	25	26	27	28
29	30	31				

Fatigue Tracker

Fatigue is rated on a 1-5 chart with 1 being the mildest and 5 being the worst. Note any specific insomnia or difficulty functioning.

1	2	3	4	5	6	7
8	9	10	11	12	13	14
15	16	17	18	19	20	21
22	23	24	25	26	27	28
29	30	31				

Mood Tracker

Mood Key:
1._____   2._____   3._____   4._____
5._____

1	2	3	4	5	6	7
8	9	10	11	12	13	14
15	16	17	18	19	20	21
22	23	24	25	26	27	28
29	30	31				

Doctor's Appointment Notes:

Date:

Doctor's Name:

Symptoms to Discuss:	Questions for the Doctor:

Notes from the Appointment:

Doctor's Appointment Notes:

Date:

Doctor's Name:

Symptoms to Discuss:	Questions for the Doctor:

Notes from the Appointment:

Doctor's Appointment Notes:

Date:

Doctor's Name:

Symptoms to Discuss:

Questions for the Doctor:

Notes from the Appointment:

Doctor's Appointment Notes:

Date:

Doctor's Name:

Symptoms to Discuss:

Questions for the Doctor:

Notes from the Appointment:

Doctor's Appointment Notes:

Date:

Doctor's Name:

Symptoms to Discuss:

Questions for the Doctor:

Notes from the Appointment:

Doctor's Appointment Notes:

Date:

Doctor's Name:

Symptoms to Discuss:

Questions for the Doctor:

Notes from the Appointment:

Doctor's Appointment Notes:

Date:

Doctor's Name:

Symptoms to Discuss:	Questions for the Doctor:

Notes from the Appointment:

Month:

Appointment Month At a Glance

Month: _____

1	
2	
3	
4	
5	
6	
7	
8	
9	
10	
11	
12	
13	
14	
15	
16	

Appointment Month At a Glance

Month: _____

17	
18	
19	
20	
21	
22	
23	
24	
25	
26	
27	
28	
29	
30	
31	

Pain Tracker

Pain is rated on a 1-5 chart with 1 being the mildest and 5 being the worst. Note any specific pain on the appropriate date.

1	2	3	4	5	6	7
8	9	10	11	12	13	14
15	16	17	18	19	20	21
22	23	24	25	26	27	28
29	30	31				

Fatigue Tracker

Fatigue is rated on a 1-5 chart with 1 being the mildest and 5 being the worst. Note any specific insomnia or difficulty functioning.

1	2	3	4	5	6	7
8	9	10	11	12	13	14
15	16	17	18	19	20	21
22	23	24	25	26	27	28
29	30	31				

Mood Tracker

Mood Key:

1._____ 2._____ 3._____ 4._____

5._____

1	2	3	4	5	6	7
8	9	10	11	12	13	14
15	16	17	18	19	20	21
22	23	24	25	26	27	28
29	30	31				

Doctor's Appointment Notes:

Date:

Doctor's Name:

Symptoms to Discuss:

Questions for the Doctor:

Notes from the Appointment:

Doctor's Appointment Notes:

Date:

Doctor's Name:

Symptoms to Discuss:	Questions for the Doctor:

Notes from the Appointment:

Doctor's Appointment Notes:

Date:

Doctor's Name:

Symptoms to Discuss:	Questions for the Doctor:

Notes from the Appointment:

Doctor's Appointment Notes:

Date:

Doctor's Name:

Symptoms to Discuss:

Questions for the Doctor:

Notes from the Appointment:

Doctor's Appointment Notes:

Date:

Doctor's Name:

Symptoms to Discuss:

Questions for the Doctor:

Notes from the Appointment:

Doctor's Appointment Notes:

Date:

Doctor's Name:

Symptoms to Discuss:	Questions for the Doctor:

Notes from the Appointment:

Doctor's Appointment Notes:

Date:

Doctor's Name:

Symptoms to Discuss:

Questions for the Doctor:

Notes from the Appointment:

Month:

Appointment Month At a Glance

Month: _____

1	
2	
3	
4	
5	
6	
7	
8	
9	
10	
11	
12	
13	
14	
15	
16	

Appointment Month At a Glance

Month: _____

17	
18	
19	
20	
21	
22	
23	
24	
25	
26	
27	
28	
29	
30	
31	

Pain Tracker

Pain is rated on a 1-5 chart with 1 being the mildest and 5 being the worst. Note any specific pain on the appropriate date.

1	2	3	4	5	6	7
8	9	10	11	12	13	14
15	16	17	18	19	20	21
22	23	24	25	26	27	28
29	30	31				

Fatigue Tracker

Fatigue is rated on a 1-5 chart with 1 being the mildest and 5 being the worst. Note any specific insomnia or difficulty functioning.

1	2	3	4	5	6	7
8	9	10	11	12	13	14
15	16	17	18	19	20	21
22	23	24	25	26	27	28
29	30	31				

Mood Tracker

Mood Key:

1._____ 2. _____ 3. _____ 4._____

5._____

1	2	3	4	5	6	7
8	9	10	11	12	13	14
15	16	17	18	19	20	21
22	23	24	25	26	27	28
29	30	31				

Doctor's Appointment Notes:

Date:

Doctor's Name:

Symptoms to Discuss:	Questions for the Doctor:

Notes from the Appointment:

Doctor's Appointment Notes:

Date:

Doctor's Name:

Symptoms to Discuss:

Questions for the Doctor:

Notes from the Appointment:

Doctor's Appointment Notes:

Date:

Doctor's Name:

Symptoms to Discuss:

Questions for the Doctor:

Notes from the Appointment:

Doctor's Appointment Notes:

Date:

Doctor's Name:

Symptoms to Discuss:	Questions for the Doctor:

Notes from the Appointment:

Doctor's Appointment Notes:

Date:

Doctor's Name:

Symptoms to Discuss:

Questions for the Doctor:

Notes from the Appointment:

Doctor's Appointment Notes:

Date:

Doctor's Name:

Symptoms to Discuss:

Questions for the Doctor:

Notes from the Appointment:

Doctor's Appointment Notes:

Date:

Doctor's Name:

Symptoms to Discuss:	Questions for the Doctor:

Notes from the Appointment:

Month:

Appointment Month At a Glance

Month: _____

1	
2	
3	
4	
5	
6	
7	
8	
9	
10	
11	
12	
13	
14	
15	
16	

Appointment Month At a Glance

Month: _____

17	
18	
19	
20	
21	
22	
23	
24	
25	
26	
27	
28	
29	
30	
31	

Pain Tracker

Pain is rated on a 1-5 chart with 1 being the mildest and 5 being the worst. Note any specific pain on the appropriate date.

1	2	3	4	5	6	7
8	9	10	11	12	13	14
15	16	17	18	19	20	21
22	23	24	25	26	27	28
29	30	31				

Fatigue Tracker

Fatigue is rated on a 1-5 chart with 1 being the mildest and 5 being the worst. Note any specific insomnia or difficulty functioning.

1	2	3	4	5	6	7
8	9	10	11	12	13	14
15	16	17	18	19	20	21
22	23	24	25	26	27	28
29	30	31				

Mood Tracker

Mood Key:

1._____ 2. _____ 3. _____ 4._____

5._____

1	2	3	4	5	6	7
8	9	10	11	12	13	14
15	16	17	18	19	20	21
22	23	24	25	26	27	28
29	30	31				

Doctor's Appointment Notes:

Date:

Doctor's Name:

Symptoms to Discuss:	Questions for the Doctor:

Notes from the Appointment:

Doctor's Appointment Notes:

Date:

Doctor's Name:

Symptoms to Discuss:

Questions for the Doctor:

Notes from the Appointment:

Doctor's Appointment Notes:

Date:

Doctor's Name:

Symptoms to Discuss:	Questions for the Doctor:

Notes from the Appointment:

Doctor's Appointment Notes:

Date:

Doctor's Name:

Symptoms to Discuss:

Questions for the Doctor:

Notes from the Appointment:

Doctor's Appointment Notes:

Date:

Doctor's Name:

Symptoms to Discuss:	Questions for the Doctor:

Notes from the Appointment:

Doctor's Appointment Notes:

Date:

Doctor's Name:

Symptoms to Discuss:

Questions for the Doctor:

Notes from the Appointment:

Doctor's Appointment Notes:

Date:

Doctor's Name:

Symptoms to Discuss:	Questions for the Doctor:

Notes from the Appointment:

Month:

Appointment Month At a Glance

Month: _____

1	
2	
3	
4	
5	
6	
7	
8	
9	
10	
11	
12	
13	
14	
15	
16	

Appointment Month At a Glance

Month: _____

17	
18	
19	
20	
21	
22	
23	
24	
25	
26	
27	
28	
29	
30	
31	

Pain Tracker

Pain is rated on a 1-5 chart with 1 being the mildest and 5 being the worst. Note any specific pain on the appropriate date.

1	2	3	4	5	6	7
8	9	10	11	12	13	14
15	16	17	18	19	20	21
22	23	24	25	26	27	28
29	30	31				

Fatigue Tracker

Fatigue is rated on a 1-5 chart with 1 being the mildest and 5 being the worst. Note any specific insomnia or difficulty functioning.

1	2	3	4	5	6	7
8	9	10	11	12	13	14
15	16	17	18	19	20	21
22	23	24	25	26	27	28
29	30	31				

Mood Tracker

Mood Key:

1._____ 2._____ 3._____ 4._____

5._____

1	2	3	4	5	6	7
8	9	10	11	12	13	14
15	16	17	18	19	20	21
22	23	24	25	26	27	28
29	30	31				

Doctor's Appointment Notes:

Date:

Doctor's Name:

Symptoms to Discuss:	Questions for the Doctor:

Notes from the Appointment:

Doctor's Appointment Notes:

Date:

Doctor's Name:

Symptoms to Discuss:

Questions for the Doctor:

Notes from the Appointment:

Doctor's Appointment Notes:

Date:

Doctor's Name:

Symptoms to Discuss:

Questions for the Doctor:

Notes from the Appointment:

Doctor's Appointment Notes:

Date:

Doctor's Name:

Symptoms to Discuss:

Questions for the Doctor:

Notes from the Appointment:

Doctor's Appointment Notes:

Date:

Doctor's Name:

Symptoms to Discuss:	Questions for the Doctor:

Notes from the Appointment:

Doctor's Appointment Notes:

Date:

Doctor's Name:

Symptoms to Discuss:

Questions for the Doctor:

Notes from the Appointment:

Doctor's Appointment Notes:

Date:

Doctor's Name:

Symptoms to Discuss:

Questions for the Doctor:

Notes from the Appointment:

www.ingramcontent.com/pod-product-compliance
Lightning Source LLC
Chambersburg PA
CBHW080544220526
45466CB00010B/3026